Disclaimer Notice:

Please note the information contained within this document is for educational and entertainment purposes only. All effort has been executed to present accurate, up to date, and reliable, complete information. No warranties of any kind are declared or implied. Readers acknowledge that the author is not engaging in the rendering of legal, financial, medical or professional advice. The content within this book has been derived from various sources. Please consult a licensed professional before attempting any techniques outlined in this book.

By reading this document, the reader agrees that under no circumstances is the author responsible for any losses, direct or indirect, which are incurred as a result of the use of information contained within this document, including, but not limited to, — errors, omissions, or inaccuracies

Table of Content

Breakfast

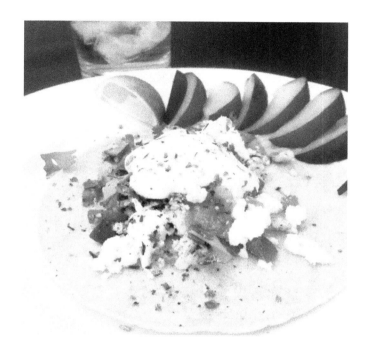

Thai Chicken Noodle Soup

Preparation Time: 10 minutes

Cooking Time: 10 minutes

Servings: 2-3

Ingredients:

- 6 cups low-sodium chicken broth
- 1-2 fresh chicken breasts, chopped
- 1 stalk lemongrass, minced
- 1 bay leaf
- 1 tablespoon ginger, grated
- 1 large carrot, sliced
- 1 cup broccoli florets, trimmed
- 1 cup mushrooms, quartered
- 1/2 teaspoon. Cayenne pepper
- 3 cloves garlic, minced
- 1/4 cup fresh lime juice
- 2 Tablespoon. Gluten-free soy sauce
- 1/4 cup coconut almond milk
- Salt and black pepper (to taste)
- A handful of fresh cilantro, chopped
- 8-10 oz. gluten-free flat Thai rice noodles

Directions:

1. Boil noodles according to package directions, or until al dente. Drain and set aside.

2. Pour chicken broth in a large pot and bring to a boil over high heat. Add chicken, broccoli, mushrooms,

lemongrass, ginger, carrot, bay leaf. Turn heat to high and allow the broth to boil for 1 minute. Cover the pot and reduce heat to medium. Simmer the soup for 6 more minutes.

3.   While the soup is simmering, stir in cayenne, garlic, lime juice, and soy sauce. Turn heat to low and add the coconut almond milk; stir well.

4.   Place cooked noodles into bowls. Pour soup over the noodles, then sprinkle with cilantro.

Nutrition: Calories: 503 kcal Protein: 48.11 g Fat: 19.63 g Carbohydrates: 35.9 g

Wedding Soup

Preparation Time: 15 minutes

Cooking Time: 60 minutes

Servings: 6

Ingredients:

- 3 slices Italian bread, toasted
- ¾ pound lean ground beef
- 1 egg or ¼ cup egg substitute
- 1 yellow onion, chopped
- 3 cloves garlic, minced
- ¼ bunch fresh parsley, chopped
- 3 sprigs fresh oregano, chopped
- 2 sprigs fresh basil, chopped
- Freshly cracked black pepper, to taste
- 4 ounces fresh grated Parmesan cheese
- 1 cup rough chopped fresh spinach with stems removed
- 2 quarts Rich Poultry Stock or low-sodium canned chicken stock

Directions:

1. Preheat oven to 375°F.

2. Wet the toasted Italian bread with water, then squeeze out all the liquid.

3. In a big bowl, mix together the bread, beef, egg, onion, garlic, parsley, oregano, basil, pepper, and half of the Parmesan. Form the mixture into 1- to 2-inch balls; place in a

baking dish and cook for 20 to 30 minutes. Take off from the oven and drain on paper towels.

4.   Steam the spinach al dente. In a large stockpot, combine the stock, spinach, and meatballs; simmer for 30 minutes.

5.   Spoon the soup into serving bowls then top with the remaining cheese

Nutrition: Calories: 245 Fat: 10 g Protein: 26 g Sodium: 1,021 mg Fiber: 0.5 g Carbohydrate: 9 g

Creamy Pumpkin Soup

Preparation time: 10 minutes

Cooking time: 20 minutes

Servings: 4

Ingredients:

- 1 onion, chopped
- 1 slice of bacon
- 2 tsp ground ginger
- 1 tsp cinnamon
- 1 cup applesauce
- 3 ½ cups low sodium chicken broth
- 1 29-oz can pumpkin
- Pepper to taste
- ½ cup light sour cream

Directions:

1. On medium high fire, place a soup pot and add bacon once hot. Sauté until crispy, around 4 minutes. Discard bacon fat, before continuing to cook. Add ginger, applesauce, chicken broth and pumpkin. Lightly season with pepper. Bring to a simmer and cook for 11 minutes. Taste and adjust seasoning. Turn off fire, stir in sour cream and mix well.

Nutrition: calories 220, fat 8 g, fiber 10 g, carbs 36 g, protein 10 g

Harvest Stew

Preparation Time: 15 minutes

Cooking Time: 60 minutes

Servings: 6

Ingredients:

- 1 pound stewing beef cubes
- 2 tablespoons olive oil
- ¼ cup flour
- ¾ cup diced onions
- ½ cup sliced carrots
- ½ cup diced celery
- 1 leek, cleaned and diced
- 6 garlic cloves, peeled
- 2 cups diced zucchini
- 1 potato, peeled and diced
- 3 turnips, diced
- 2 bell pepper, chopped
- 1 bay leaf
- 3 sprigs fresh thyme
- 4 cups low-sodium beef broth
- 2 tablespoons Worcestershire sauce
- Salt and pepper, to taste

Directions:

1. Brown the beef cubes in olive oil. Dust the flour on the meat and stir to coat and distribute.

2.   Add the onions, carrots, celery, leek, garlic, zucchini, potato, turnips, bell pepper, bay leaf, thyme sprigs, and beef broth. Place to a boil, then lower the heat and simmer for 60 minutes.

3.   Remove the bay leaf and thyme sprigs. Add the Worcestershire sauce, salt, and pepper. Serve hot.

Nutrition: Calories: 254 Fat: 9.5 g Protein: 20 g Sodium: 514 mg Fiber: 3.5 g Carbohydrate: 22 g

Mediterranean Stew

Preparation Time: 10 minutes

Cooking Time: 15 minutes

Servings: 4

Ingredients:

- 3 tablespoons olive oil
- 3 cloves garlic, crushed and minced
- 1 (15½-ounce) can chickpeas, drained and rinsed
- 1 (19-ounce) can cannellini beans, drained and rinsed
- 2 cups roasted bell pepper
- 1½ cups artichoke hearts, quartered
- 1 cup Basic Vegetable Stock or low-sodium canned vegetable stock
- 4 tablespoons grated Parmesan cheese
- 1 teaspoon red pepper, crushed or to taste
- 1 teaspoon dried oregano
- Salt, to taste
- Freshly ground black pepper, to taste
- Chopped sun-dried bell pepper, for garnish
- Chopped Italian parsley, for garnish
- Garlic-seasoned croutons, for garnish
- Crumbled feta cheese, for garnish
- Fresh oregano leaves, for garnish

Directions:

1.   Warm the olive oil in a huge saucepan on medium heat and sauté the garlic for 2 to 3 minutes or until golden.

2.   Reduce the heat to medium-low. Stir in the chickpeas, cannellini beans, roasted bell pepper, artichoke hearts, stock, Parmesan cheese, crushed red pepper, oregano, salt, and pepper. Cook and stir for about 10 minutes. Serve in individual bowls, garnishing as desired.

Nutrition: Calories: 445 Fat: 16 g Protein: 18 g Sodium: 530 mg Fiber: 12 g Carbohydrate: 61 g

Chicken and Pasta Salad

Preparation time: 30 minutes

Cooking time: 25 minutes

Servings: 6

Ingredients:

- Chicken Pasta Salad
- 6 oz. cooked chicken
- 3 - cups pasta, spiral, cooked
- ½ - green pepper, minced
- 1 ½ - tbsp. onion
- ½ - cup celery
- Garlic Mustard Vinaigrette
- 2 - tbsp. cider Vinegar
- 2 - tsp mustard, prepared
- ½ - tsp. white sugar
- 1 - garlic clove, Minced
- 1/3 - cup water
- 1/3 - cup olive oil
- 2 - tsp. parmesan cheese, grated
- ½ - tsp. ground pepper

Directions:

1.   In a little bowl, combine vinegar, mustard, sugar, garlic, and water; slowly race in oil.

2.   Mix in Parmesan. Season with pepper.

3.   Join 1⁄3 measure of dressing with Chicken Pasta Salad and chill.

Nutrition: Calories 233, fat 12 g, fiber 6g, carbs 25 g, protein 23 g

Garlic Cauliflower Rice

Preparation Time: 10 minutes

Cooking Time: 5 minutes

Servings: 8

Ingredients:

- 1 medium head cauliflower
- 1 tablespoon extra-virgin olive oil
- 4 garlic cloves, minced
- Freshly ground black pepper

Directions:

1. Using a sharp knife, remove the core of the cauliflower, and separate the cauliflower into florets.

2. In a food processor, pulse the florets until they are the size of rice, being careful not to over process them to the point of becoming mushy.

3. In a large skillet over medium heat, heat the olive oil. Add the garlic, and stir until just fragrant.

4. Add the cauliflower, stirring to coat. Add 1 tablespoon of water to the pan, cover, and reduce the heat to low. Steam for 7 to 10 minutes, until the cauliflower is tender. Season with pepper and serve.

Nutrition: Calories: 37; Total Fat: 2g; Saturated Fat: 0g; Cholesterol: 0mg; Carbohydrates: 4g; Fiber: 2g; Protein: 2g; Phosphorus: 35mg; Potassium: 226mg; Sodium: 22mg

Creamy Broccoli Soup

Preparation Time: 10 minutes

Cooking Time: 15 minutes

Servings: 4

Ingredients:

- 1 teaspoon extra-virgin olive oil
- ½ sweet onion, roughly chopped
- 2 cups chopped broccoli
- 4 cups low-sodium vegetable broth
- Freshly ground black pepper
- 1 cup Homemade Rice Almond milk or unsweetened store-bought rice almond milk
- ¼ cup grated Parmesan cheese

Directions:

1. Heat the olive oil. Add the onion and cook for 3 to 5 minutes, until it begins to soften. Add the broccoli and broth, and season with pepper.

2. Bring to a boil, reduce the heat, and simmer open for 10 minutes, until the broccoli is just tender but still bright green.

3. Transfer the soup mixture to a blender. Add the rice almond milk, and process until smooth. Return to the saucepan, stir in the Parmesan cheese, and serve.

Nutrition: Calories: 88; Total Fat: 3g; Saturated Fat: 1g; Cholesterol: 6mg; Carbohydrates: 12g; Fiber: 3g; Protein: 4g; Phosphorus: 87mg; Potassium: 201mg; Sodium: 281mg

Curried Carrot and Beet Soup

Preparation Time: 10 minutes

Cooking Time: 50 minutes

Servings: 4

Ingredients:

*   1 large red beet
*   5 carrots, chopped
*   1 tablespoon curry powder
*   3 cups Homemade Rice Almond milk or unsweetened store-bought rice almond milk
*   Freshly ground black pepper
*   Yogurt, for serving

Directions:

1.   Preheat the oven to 400°F.

2.   Wrap the beet in aluminum foil and roast for 45 minutes, until the vegetable is tender when pierced with a fork. Remove from the oven and let cool.

3.   Add the carrots and cover with water. Bring to a boil, reduce the heat, cover, and simmer for 10 minutes, until tender.

4.   Transfer the carrots and beet to a food processor, and process until smooth. Add the curry powder and rice almond milk. Season with pepper. Serve topped with a dollop of yogurt.

5.   Substitution tip: Carrots are high in potassium. If you need to reduce your potassium further, use 2 carrots instead of

5. The soup will be a little thinner but still have a carrot flavor and just 322mg of potassium.

Nutrition: Calories: 112; Total Fat: 1g; Saturated Fat: 0g; Cholesterol: 0mg; Carbohydrates: 24g; Fiber: 7g; Protein: 3g; Phosphorus: 57mg; Potassium: 468mg; Sodium: 129mg

Coconut Curried Ban-Apple Soup

Preparation Time: 10 minutes

Cooking Time: 10-15 minutes

Servings: 4

Ingredients:

- 2 cups Basic Vegetable Stock or low-sodium canned vegetable stock
- 1 ripe banana
- 1 large potato 1 Granny Smith apple
- 1 celery heart
- 1 sweet onion
- 1 cup coconut almond milk
- 1 teaspoon curry powder
- 1 teaspoon salt
- ¼ cup toasted coconut, for garnish
- 2 tablespoons chopped fresh cilantro, for garnish

Directions:

1. Put the vegetable stock in a soup pot.

2. Peel the banana and potato, chop them, and put them in the soup pot. Core the apple, chop it, and add it to the soup pot. Chop the celery heart and onion and add them to the soup pot.

3. Place the soup to a boil, then lower the heat and simmer for 10 to 15 minutes. Add the coconut almond milk, curry powder, and salt.

4. Put the hot soup in a blender and purée.

5.　　Serve the soup hot. Garnish with toasted coconut and cilantro.

Nutrition: Calories: 344 Fat: 19 g Protein: 6 g Sodium: 886 mg Fiber: 7 g Carbohydrate: 40 g

Herbed Soup with Black Beans

Preparation time: 10 minutes

Cooking time: 10 minutes

Servings: 4

Ingredients:

- 2 tbsp tomato paste
- 1/3 cup Poblano pepper, charred, peeled, seeded and chopped
- 2 cups vegetable stock
- ¼ tsp cumin
- ½ tsp paprika
- ½ tsp dried oregano
- 2 tsp fresh garlic, minced
- 1 cup onion, small diced
- 1 tbsp extra-virgin olive oil
- 1 15-oz can black beans, drained and rinsed

Directions:

1. On medium fire, place a soup pot and heat oil. Add onion and sauté until translucent and soft, around 4-5 minutes. Add garlic, cook for 2 minutes. Add the rest of the ingredients and bring to a simmer. Once simmering, turn off the fire and transfer to a blender. Puree ingredients until smooth.

Nutrition: calories 98, fat 21 g, fiber 10 g, carbs 20 g, protein 19 g

Golden Beet Soup

Preparation Time: 10 minutes

Cooking Time: 35 minutes

Servings: 4

Ingredients:

- 3 tablespoons unsalted butter
- 4 golden beets, cut into ½-inch cubes
- ½ sweet onion, chopped
- 1-inch piece ginger, minced
- Zest and juice of 1 lemon
- 4 cups Simple Chicken Broth or low-sodium store-bought chicken stock
- Freshly ground black pepper
- ¼ cup pomegranate seeds, for serving
- ¼ cup crème fraiche, for serving (see Substitution tip)
- 10 sage leaves, for serving

Directions:

1. In a medium saucepan over medium heat, melt the butter.

2. Add the beets, onion, ginger, and lemon zest, and cover. Cook, stirring occasionally, for 15 minutes. Add the broth, and continue to cook for 20 more minutes, until the beets are very tender.

3. In batches, transfer the soup to a blender and purée, or use an immersion blender.

4.   Return the soup to the saucepan, and season with the pepper and lemon juice.

5.   Serve topped with the pomegranate seeds, crème fraîche, and sage leaves.

6.   Substitution tip: You can buy crème fraîche at many grocery stores, or make your own. If you don't have crème fraîche, a dollop of whole-almond milk yogurt is a fine substitute.

Nutrition: Calories: 186; Total Fat: 11g; Saturated Fat: 7g; Cholesterol: 26mg; Carbohydrates: 17g; Fiber: 3g; Protein: 7g; Phosphorus: 125mg; Potassium: 557mg; Sodium: 148mg

Broccoli Soup with Gorgonzola Cheese

Preparation Time: 10 minutes

Cooking Time: 30 minutes

Servings: 4

Ingredients:

- 1 large broccoli, divided into small roses
- 2 carrots, peeled and diced
- 5 garlic cloves, chopped
- 1 onion, diced
- 1 tablespoon of oil
- 750 ml broth
- 1 flat teaspoon of sweet pepper
- 1 tablespoon of chopped parsley
- 1 tablespoon of chopped fresh basil
- A pinch of sugar
- 150 g Gorgonzola cheese, diced
- 1/2 cup 18% cream
- Salt and pepper
- 4 tablespoons of almond flakes roasted in a dry pan
- Pumpkin oil (optional)

Directions:

1. In a big saucepan, warm the oil on medium heat, put the onion and garlic, and fry it until the vitrified glass onion.

2. Then put the broccoli with carrots, pour the broth and cook for about 15-20 minutes until the vegetables soften. Add basil, parsley, sugar, pepper, and pepper to taste.

3.   Add cheese and cream, and when the cheese dissolves, blend with a blender until smooth. Season with salt and pepper if necessary.

4.   Serve the soup sprinkled with almond flakes and sprinkled with pumpkin oil.

Nutrition: Calories: 382 kcal Protein: 13.06 g Fat: 18.93 g Carbohydrates: 41.65 g

Cauliflower and Chive Soup

Preparation Time: 10 minutes

Cooking Time: 20 minutes

Servings: 4

Ingredients:

- 2 tablespoons extra-virgin olive oil
- ½ sweet onion, chopped
- 2 garlic cloves, minced
- 2 cups Simple Chicken Broth or low-sodium store-bought chicken stock
- 1 cauliflower head, broken into florets
- Freshly ground black pepper
- 4 tablespoons (¼ cup) finely chopped chives

Directions:

1.   Heat the olive oil.

2.   Add the onion and cook, stirring frequently, for 3 to 5 minutes, until it begins to soften. Add the garlic and stir until fragrant.

3.   Add the broth and cauliflower, and bring to a boil. Reduce the heat and simmer until the cauliflower is tender, about 15 minutes.

4.   Transfer the soup in batches to a blender or food processor and purée until smooth, or use an immersion blender.

5. Return the soup to the pot, and season with pepper. Before serving, top each bowl with 1 tablespoon of chives.

Nutrition: Calories 132; Total Fat: 8g; Saturated Fat: 1g; Cholesterol: 0mg; Carbohydrates: 13g; Fiber: 3g;Protein: 6g; Phosphorus: 116mg; Potassium: 607mg; Sodium: 84mg

Cauliflower Soup

Preparation Time: 15 minutes

Cooking Time: 10 minutes

Servings: 4

Ingredients:

- Unsalted butter – 1 tsp.
- Sweet onion – 1 small, chopped
- Minced garlic – 2 tsps.
- Small head cauliflower – 1, cut into small florets
- Curry powder – 2 tsps.
- Water to cover the cauliflower
- Light sour cream – ½ cup
- Chopped fresh cilantro – 3 Tbsps.

Directions:

1. Heat the butter over a medium-high heat and sauté the onion-garlic for about 3 minutes or until softened.

2. Add the cauliflower, water, and curry powder.

3. Bring the soup to a simmer, then decrease the heat to low and simmer for 20 minutes or until the cauliflower is tender.

4. Puree the soup until creamy and smooth with a hand mixer.

5. Transfer the soup back into a saucepan and stir in the sour cream and cilantro.

6.   Heat the soup on medium heat for 5 minutes or until warmed through.

Nutrition: Calories: 33 Fat: 2g Carb: 4g Phosphorus: 30mg Potassium: 167mg Sodium: 22mg Protein: 1g

Leek, and Carrot Soup

Preparation time: 15 minutes

Cooking time: 25 minutes

Servings: 4

Ingredients:

*   1 - Leek
*   ¾ - cup diced and boiled carrots
*   1 - Garlic clove
*   1 - tbsp. oil
*   Crushed pepper to taste
*   3 - Cups low sodium chicken stock
*   Chopped parsley for garnish
*   1 - Bay leaf
*   ¼ - tsp. ground cumin

Directions:

1.   Trim off and take away a portion of the coarse inexperienced portions of the leek, at that factor reduce daintily and flush altogether in virus water. Channel properly. Warmth the oil in an extensively based pot. Include the leek and garlic, and sear over low warmth for two-3 minutes, till sensitive. Include the inventory, inlet leaf, cumin, and pepper.

2.   Heat the mixture to the point of boiling, mixing constantly. Include carrots and stew for 13 minutes. Modify the flavoring, eliminate the inlet leaf and serve sprinkled with slashed parsley. To make a pureed soup, manner the soup in a blender or nourishment processor till smooth. Come again to

the pan. Include ½ field almond milk. Bring to bubble and stew for 4 mins.

Nutrition: Calories 325, Fat 9, Fiber 5, Carbs 16, Protein 29

Creamy Vinaigrette

Preparation time: 15 minutes

Cooking time: 25 minutes

Servings: 4

Ingredients:

- 2 - tbsp. cider vinegar
- 2 - tbsp. lime or lemon juice
- 1 - garlic clove, minced
- 1 - tsp. Dijon mustard
- 1 - tsp. ground cumin
- ½ - cup sour cream
- 2 - tbsp. olive oil
- ¼ - tsp. black pepper

Directions:

1. Consolidate all fixings and blend well. Fill serving of mixed greens carafe. Chill.

Nutrition: Calories 188, fat 15, fiber 8, carbs 35, protein 25

Lunch

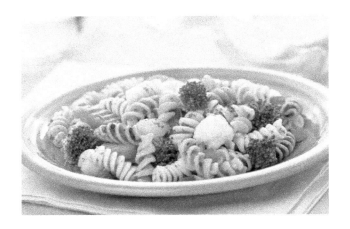

Pesto Pasta Salad

Preparation Time: 15 minutes

Cooking Time: 15 minutes

Servings: 4

Ingredients:

- 1 cup fresh basil leaves
- ½ cup packed fresh flat-leaf parsley leaves
- ½ cup arugula, chopped
- 2 tablespoons Parmesan cheese, grated
- ¼ cup extra-virgin olive oil
- 3 tablespoons mayonnaise
- 2 tablespoons water
- 12 ounces whole-wheat rotini pasta
- 1 red bell pepper, chopped
- 1 medium yellow summer squash, sliced
- 1 cup frozen baby peas

Directions:

1. Boil water in a large pot.

2. Meanwhile, combine the basil, parsley, arugula, cheese, and olive oil in a blender or food processor. Process until the herbs are finely chopped. Add the mayonnaise and water, then process again. Set aside.

3. Prepare the pasta to the pot of boiling water; cook according to package directions, about 8 to 9 minutes. Drain well, reserving ¼ cup of the cooking liquid.

4.	Combine the pesto, pasta, bell pepper, squash, and peas in a large bowl and toss gently, adding enough reserved pasta cooking liquid to make a sauce on the salad. Serve immediately or cover and chill, then serve.

5.	Store covered in the refrigerator for up to 3 days.

Nutrition: Calories: 378 Fat: 24g Carbohydrates: 35g Protein: 9g Sodium: 163mg Potassium: 472mg Phosphorus: 213mg

Creamy Shells with Peas and Bacon

Preparation Time: 15 minutes

Cooking Time: 15 minutes

Servings: 4

Ingredients:

- 1 cup part-skim ricotta cheese
- ½ cup grated Parmesan cheese
- 3 slices bacon, cut into strips
- 1 cup onion, chopped
- ¾ cup of frozen green peas
- 1 tbsp. olive oil
- ¼ tsp black pepper
- 3 garlic cloves, minced
- 3 cup cooked whole-wheat small shell pasta
- 1 tbsp. lemon juice
- 2 tbsp. unsalted butter

Directions:

1. Place ricotta, Parmesan cheese, butter, and pepper in a large bowl.
2. Cook bacon in a skillet until crisp. Set aside.
3. Add the garlic and onion to the same skillet and fry until soft. Add to bowl with ricotta.
4. Cook the peas and add to the ricotta.
5. Add half a cup of the reserved cooking water and lemon juice to the ricotta mixture and mix well.

6.   Add the pasta, bacon, and peas to the bowl and mix well.

7.   Put freshly ground black pepper and serve.

Nutrition: Calories 429 Fat 14g Carbs 27g Protein 13g Sodium 244mg Potassium 172mg Phosphorous 203mg

Egg and Veggie Fajitas

Preparation Time: 15 minutes

Cooking Time: 10 minutes

Servings: 4

Ingredients:

- 3 large eggs
- 3 egg whites
- 2 teaspoons chili powder
- 1 tablespoon unsalted butter
- 1 onion, chopped
- 2 garlic cloves, minced
- 1 jalapeño pepper, minced
- 1 red bell pepper, chopped
- 1 cup frozen corn, thawed and drained
- 8 (6-inch) corn tortillas

Directions:

1. Whisk the eggs, egg whites, and chili powder in a small bowl until well combined. Set aside.

2. Prepare a large skillet and melt the butter on medium heat.

3. Sauté the onion, garlic, jalapeño, bell pepper, and corn until the vegetables are tender, 3 to 4 minutes.

4. Add the beaten egg mixture to the skillet. Cook, occasionally stirring, until the eggs form large curds and are set, 3 to 5 minutes.

5.   Meanwhile, soften the corn tortillas as directed on the package.

6.   Divide the egg mixture evenly among the softened corn tortillas. Roll the tortillas up and serve.

Nutrition: Calories: 316 Fat 14g Carbohydrates: 35g Protein: 14g Sodium: 167mg Potassium: 408mg Phosphorus: 287mg

Fast Cabbage Cakes

Preparation Time: 15 minutes

Cooking Time: 10 minutes

Servings: 2

Ingredients:

- 1 cup cauliflower, shredded
- 1 egg, beaten
- 1 teaspoon salt
- 1 teaspoon ground black pepper
- 2 tablespoons almond flour
- 1 teaspoon olive oil

Directions:

1. Blend the shredded cabbage in the blender until you get cabbage rice.

2. Then, mix up cabbage rice with the egg, salt, ground black pepper, and almond flour.

3. Pour olive oil in the skillet and preheat it.

4. Then make the small cakes with the help of 2 spoons and place them in the hot oil.

5. Roast the cabbage cakes for 4 minutes from each side over the medium-low heat.

Nutrition: Calories 227, Fat 18.6, Fiber 4.5, Carbs 9.5, Protein 9.9

Vegetable Biryani

Preparation Time: 10 minutes

Cooking Time: 15 minutes

Servings: 4

Ingredients:

- 2 tablespoons olive oil
- 1 onion, diced
- 4 garlic cloves, minced
- 1 tbsp. peeled and grated fresh ginger root
- 1 cup carrot, grated
- 2 cups chopped cauliflower
- 1 cup thawed frozen baby peas
- 2 teaspoons curry powder
- 1 cup low-sodium vegetable broth
- 3 cups of frozen cooked white rice

Directions:

1. Get a skillet and heat the olive oil on medium heat.

2. Add onion, garlic, and ginger root. Sauté, frequently stirring, until tender-crisp, 2 minutes.

3. Add the carrot, cauliflower, peas, and curry powder and cook for 2 minutes longer.

4. Put vegetable broth. Cover the skillet partially, and simmer on low for 6 to 7 minutes or until the vegetables are tender.

5. Meanwhile, heat the rice as directed on the package.

6.   Stir the rice into the vegetable mixture and serve.

Nutrition: Calories: 378 Fat 16g Carbohydrates: 53g Protein: 8g Sodium: 113mg Potassium: 510mg Phosphorus: 236mg

Cilantro Chili Burgers

Preparation Time: 10 minutes

Cooking Time: 15 minutes

Servings: 3

Ingredients:

- 1 cup red cabbage
- 3 tablespoons almond flour
- 1 tablespoon cream cheese
- 1 oz. scallions, chopped
- ½ teaspoon salt
- ½ teaspoon chili powder
- ½ cup fresh cilantro

Directions:

1. Chop red cabbage roughly and transfer in the blender.

2. Add fresh cilantro and blend the mixture until very smooth.

3. After this, transfer it in the bowl.

4. Add cream cheese, scallions, salt, chili powder, and almond flour.

5. Stir the mixture well.

6. Make 3 big burgers from the cabbage mixture or 6 small burgers.

7. Line the baking tray with baking paper.

8. Place the burgers in the tray.

9. Bake the cilantro burgers for 15 minutes at 360F.

10.   Flip the burgers onto another side after 8 minutes of cooking.

Nutrition: Calories 182, Fat 15.3, Fiber 4.1, Carbs 8.5, Protein 6.8

Double-Boiled Stewed Carrots

Preparation Time: 20 minutes

Cooking Time: 30 minutes

Servings: 4

Ingredients:

- 2 cup carrots, diced into ½ inch cubes
- ½ cup hot water
- ½ cup liquid non-dairy creamer
- ¼ tsp garlic powder
- ¼ tsp black pepper
- 2 tbsp. margarine
- 2 tsp all-purpose white flour

Directions:

1. Soak or double boil the carrots if you are on a low potassium diet.

2. Boil carrots for 15 minutes.

3. Drain carrots and return to pan. Add half a cup of hot water, the creamer, garlic powder, pepper, and margarine. Heat to a boil.

4. Mix the flour with a tablespoon of water and then stir this into the carrots. Cook for 3 minutes until the mixture has thickened and the flour has cooked.

Nutrition: Calories 184 Carbs 25g Protein 2g Potassium 161mg Phosphorous 65mg

24. Double-Boiled Country Style Fried Carrots

Preparation Time: 20 minutes

Cooking Time: 20 minutes

Servings: 4

Ingredients:

- ½ cup canola oil
- ¼ tsp ground cumin
- ¼ tsp paprika
- ¼ tsp white pepper
- 3 tbsp. ketchup

Directions:

1. Soak or double boil the carrots if you are on a low potassium diet.

2. Heat oil over medium heat in a skillet.

3. Fry the carrots for around 10 minutes until golden brown.

4. Drain carrots, then sprinkle with cumin, pepper, and paprika.

5. Serve with ketchup or mayo.

Nutrition: Calories 156 Fat 0.1g Carbs 21g Protein 2g Sodium 3mg Potassium 296mg Phosphorous 34mg

Broccoli-Onion Latkes

Preparation Time: 15 minutes

Cooking Time: 20 minutes

Servings: 4

Ingredients:

- 3 cups broccoli florets, diced
- ½ cup onion, chopped
- 2 large eggs, beaten
- 2 tbsp. all-purpose white flour
- 2 tbsp. olive oil

Directions:

1. Cook the broccoli for around 5 minutes until tender. Drain.

2. Mix the flour into the eggs.

3. Combine the onion, broccoli, and egg mixture and stir through.

4. Prepare olive oil in a skillet on medium-high heat.

5. Drop a spoon of the mixture onto the pan to make 4 latkes.

6. Cook each side until golden brown.

7. Drain on a paper towel and serve.

Nutrition: Calories 140 Fat Carbs 7g Protein 6g Sodium 58mg Potassium 276mg Phosphorous 101mg

Vegetable Masala

Preparation Time: 10 minutes

Cooking Time: 18 minutes

Servings: 4

Ingredients:

- 2 cups green beans, chopped
- 1 cup white mushroom, chopped
- ¾ cup Red bell peppers, crushed
- 1 teaspoon minced garlic
- 1 teaspoon minced ginger
- 1 teaspoon chili flakes
- 1 tablespoon garam masala
- 1 tablespoon olive oil
- 1 teaspoon salt

Directions:

1.   Line the tray with parchment and preheat the oven to 360F.

2.   Place the green beans and mushrooms in the tray.

3.   Sprinkle the vegetables with crushed Red bell peppers, minced garlic and ginger, chili flakes, garam masala, olive oil, and salt.

4.   Mix up well and transfer in the oven.

5.   Cook vegetable masala for 18 minutes.

Nutrition: Calories 60, Fat 30.7, Fiber 2.5, Carbs 6.4, Protein 2

Dinner

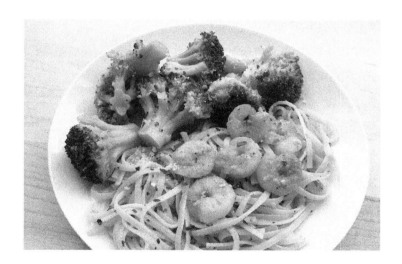

Roasted Spatchcock Chicken

Preparation Time: 20 minutes

Cooking Time: 50 minutes

Servings: 4-6

Ingredients:

- 1 (4-pound) whole chicken
- 1 (1-inch) piece fresh ginger, sliced
- 4 garlic cloves, chopped
- 1 small bunch of fresh thyme
- Pinch of cayenne
- Salt
- ground black pepper
- ¼ cup fresh lemon juice
- 3 tablespoons extra virgin olive oil

Directions:

1. Arrange chicken, breast side down onto a large cutting board. With a kitchen shear, begin with the thigh, cut along 1 side of the backbone, and turn the chicken around.

2. Now, cut along sleep issues and discard the backbone. Change the inside and open it like a book. Flatten the backbone firmly to flatten.

3. In a food processor, add all ingredients except chicken and pulse till smooth. In a big baking dish, add the marinade mixture.

4.   Add chicken and coat with marinade generously. With a plastic wrap, cover the baking dish and refrigerate to marinate overnight.

5.   Preheat the oven to 450 degrees F. Arrange a rack in a very roasting pan. Remove the chicken from the refrigerator makes onto a rack over the roasting pan, skin side down. Roast for about 50 minutes, turning once in a middle way.

Nutrition: Calories: 419 Fat: 14g Carbohydrates: 28g Protein: 40g Phosphorus 166 mg Potassium 196 mg Sodium 68 mg

Chicken Meatloaf with Veggies

Preparation Time: 20 minutes

Cooking Time: 1-1¼ hours

Servings: 4

Ingredients:

- For Meatloaf:
- ½ cup cooked chickpeas
- 2 egg whites
- 2½ teaspoons poultry seasoning
- Salt
- ground black pepper
- 10-ounce lean ground chicken
- 1 cup red bell pepper, seeded and minced
- 1 cup celery stalk, minced
- 1/3 cup steel-cut oats
- 1 cup tomato puree, divided
- 2 tablespoons dried onion flakes, crushed
- 1 tablespoon prepared mustard
- For Veggies:
- 2-pounds summer squash, sliced
- 16-ounce frozen Brussels sprouts
- 2 tablespoons extra-virgin extra virgin olive oil
- Salt
- ground black pepper

Directions:

1. Warm oven to 350 degrees F. Grease a 9x5-inch loaf pan. In a mixer, add chickpeas, egg whites, poultry seasoning, salt, and black pepper and pulse till smooth.

2. Transfer a combination in a large bowl. Add chicken, veggies oats, ½ cup of tomato puree, and onion flakes and mix till well combined.

3. Transfer the amalgamation into the prepared loaf pan evenly. With both hands, press down the amalgamation slightly.

4. In another bowl, mix mustard and remaining tomato puree. Place the mustard mixture over the loaf pan evenly.

5. Bake approximately 1-1¼ hours or till the desired doneness. Meanwhile, in a big pan of water, arrange a steamer basket. Cover and steam for about 10-12 minutes. Drain well and aside.

6. Now, prepare the Brussels sprouts according to the package's directions. In a big bowl, add veggies, oil, salt, and black pepper and toss to coat well. Serve the meatloaf with veggies.

Nutrition: Calories: 420 Fat: 9g Carbohydrates: 21g Protein: 36g Phosphorus 237.1 mg Potassium 583.6 mg Sodium 136 mg

Roasted Chicken with Veggies & Mango

Preparation Time: 20 minutes

Cooking Time: 1 hour

Servings: 4

Ingredients:

- 1 teaspoon ground ginger
- ½ teaspoon ground cumin
- ½ teaspoon ground coriander
- 1 teaspoon paprika
- Salt
- ground black pepper
- 1 (3 ½-4-pound) whole chicken
- 1 unpeeled mango, cut into 8 wedges
- 2 medium carrots, peeled and cut into 2-inch pieces
- ½ cup of water

Directions:

1. Warm oven to 450 degrees F. In a little bowl, mix the spices. Rub the chicken with spice mixture evenly.

2. Arrange the chicken in a substantial Dutch oven and put the mango, carrot, and sweet potato pieces around it.

3. Add water and cover the pan tightly. Roast for around 30 minutes. Uncover and roast for about half an hour.

Nutrition: Calories: 432 Fat: 10g Carbohydrates: 20g Protein: 34g Potassium 481 mg Sodium 418 mg Phosphorus 170 mg

Chicken & Cauliflower Rice Casserole

Preparation Time: 15 minutes

Cooking Time: 1 hour & 15 minutes

Servings: 8-10

Ingredients:

- 2 tablespoons coconut oil, divided
- 3-pound bone-in chicken thighs and drumsticks
- Salt
- ground black pepper
- 3 carrots, peeled and sliced
- 1 onion, chopped finely
- 2 garlic cloves, chopped finely
- 2 tablespoons fresh cinnamon, chopped finely
- 2 teaspoons ground cumin
- 1 teaspoon ground coriander
- 12 teaspoon ground cinnamon
- ½ teaspoon ground turmeric
- 1 teaspoon paprika
- ¼ tsp red pepper cayenne
- 1 (28-ounce) can diced Red bell peppers with liquid
- 1 red bell pepper, thin strips
- ½ cup fresh parsley leaves, minced
- Salt, to taste
- 1 head cauliflower, grated to some rice-like consistency
- 1 lemon, sliced thinly

Directions:

1.   Warm oven to 375 degrees F. In a large pan, melt 1 tablespoon of coconut oil at high heat. Add chicken pieces and cook for about 3-5 minutes per side or till golden brown.

2.   Transfer the chicken to a plate. In a similar pan, sauté the carrot, onion, garlic, and ginger for about 4-5 minutes on medium heat.

3.   Stir in spices and remaining coconut oil. Add chicken, Red bell peppers, bell pepper, parsley plus salt, and simmer for approximately 3-5 minutes.

4.   In the bottom of a 13x9-inch rectangular baking dish, spread the cauliflower rice evenly. Place chicken mixture over cauliflower rice evenly and top with lemon slices.

5.   With foil paper, cover the baking dish and bake for approximately 35 minutes. Uncover the baking dish and bake for about 25 minutes.

Nutrition: Calories: 412 Fat: 12g Carbohydrates: 23g Protein: 34g Phosphorus 201 mg Potassium 289.4 mg Sodium 507.4 mg

Poultry

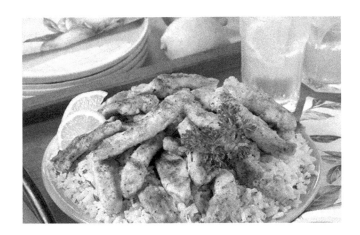

Healthy Turkey Gumbo

Preparation Time: 5 minutes

Cooking Time: 2 hours

Servings: 1

Ingredients:

- 1 Whole Turkey
- 1 Onion, quartered
- Stalk of Celery, chopped
- 3 Cloves garlic, chopped
- 1/2 cup Okra
- 1 can chopped bell pepper
- 1 tbsp. Extra virgin olive oils
- 1-2 Bay leaves
- Black pepper to taste

Directions:

1. Take the first four ingredients and add 2 cups of water in a stockpot, heating on a high heat until boiling.

2. Lower the heat and simmer for 45-50 minutes or until turkey is cooked through.

3. Remove the turkey and strain the broth.

4. Grab a skillet and then heat the oil on medium heat and brown the rest of the vegetables for 5-10 minutes.

5. Stir until tender, and then add to the broth.

6. Add the bell pepper and turkey meat to the broth and stir.

7.   Add the bay leaves and continue to cook for an hour or until the sauce has thickened.

8.   Season with black pepper and enjoy.

Nutrition: Calories: 261 kcal Protein: 11.72 g Fat: 12.91 g Carbohydrates: 28.33 g

Cauliflower and Leeks

Preparation Time: 10 minutes

Cooking Time: 20 minutes

Servings: 4

Ingredients:

- 1 and ½ cups leeks, chopped
- 1 and ½ cups cauliflower florets
- 2 garlic cloves, minced
- 1 and ½ cups artichoke hearts
- 2 tablespoons coconut oil, melted
- Black pepper to taste

Directions:

1. Heat up a pan with the oil over medium-high heat, add garlic, leeks, cauliflower florets and artichoke hearts, stir and cook for 20 minutes.

2. Add black pepper, stir, divide between plates and serve.

3. Enjoy!

Nutrition: Calories 192, fat 6,9, fiber 8,2, carbs 35,1, protein 5,1 Phosphorus: 110mg Potassium: 117mg Sodium: 75mg

Eggplant and Mushroom Sauté

Preparation Time: 10 minutes

Cooking Time: 30 minutes

Servings: 4

Ingredients:

- 2 pounds oyster mushrooms, chopped
- 6 ounces shallots, peeled, chopped
- 1 yellow onion, chopped
- 2 eggplants, cubed
- 3 celery stalks, chopped
- 1 tablespoon parsley, chopped
- A pinch of sea salt
- Black pepper to taste
- 1 tablespoon savory, dried
- 3 tablespoons coconut oil, melted

Directions:

1. Heat up a pan with the oil over medium high heat, add onion, stir and cook for 4 minutes.

2. Add shallots, stir and cook for 4 more minutes.

3. Add eggplant pieces, mushrooms, celery, savory and black pepper to taste, stir and cook for 15 minutes.

4. Add parsley, stir again, cook for a couple more minutes, divide between plates and serve.

5. Enjoy!

Nutrition: calories 1013, fat 10,9, fiber 35,5, carbs 156,5, protein 69,1 Phosphorus: 210mg Potassium: 217mg Sodium: 105mg

Chickpea Curry Soup

Preparation Time: 10 minutes

Cooking Time: 25 minutes

Servings: 4

Ingredients:

- ¼ cup extra-virgin olive oil or coconut oil
- 1 medium onion, finely chopped
- 2 garlic cloves, sliced
- 1 large apple, cored, peeled, and cut into ¼-inch dice
- 2 teaspoons curry powder
- 1 teaspoon salt
- 3 cups peeled butternut squash cut into ½-inch dice
- 3 cups vegetable broth
- 1 cup full-fat coconut almond milk
- 1 (15-ounce) can chickpeas, drained and rinsed
- 2 tablespoons finely chopped fresh cilantro

Directions:

1. In a huge pot, heat the oil on high heat.
2. Add the onion and garlic and sauté until the onion begins to brown, 6 to 8 minutes.
3. Put the apple, curry powder, and salt and sauté to toast the curry powder, 1 to 2 minutes.
4. Put the squash and broth then bring to a boil.
5. Lower the heat then cook until the squash is tender about 10 minutes.
6. Stir in the coconut almond milk.

7.   Using an immersion blender, purée the soup in the pot until smooth.

8.   Stir in the chickpeas and cilantro, heat through for 1 to 2 minutes, and serve.

Nutrition: Calories: 469 Total Fat: 30g Total Carbohydrates: 45g Sugar: 14g Fiber: 10g Protein: 12g Sodium: 1174mg

Cajun Chicken & Prawn

Preparation Time: 5 minutes

Cooking Time: 35 minutes

Servings: 2

Ingredients:

- 2 Free-range Skinless Chicken breast, chopped
- 1 Onion, chopped
- 1 Red pepper, chopped
- 2 Garlic cloves, crushed
- 10 Fresh or frozen prawn
- 1 tsp. Cayenne powder
- 1 tsp. Chili powder
- 1 tsp. Paprika
- 1/4 tsp. Chili powder
- 1 tsp. Dried oregano
- 1 tsp. Dried thyme
- 1 cup Brown or wholegrain rice
- 1 tbsp. Extra Virgin olive oil
- 1 can Bell pepper, chopped
- 2 cups Homemade chicken stock

Directions:

1. In a bowl, put all the spices and herbs then mix to form your Cajun spice mix.

2. Grab a large pan and add the olive oil, heating on medium heat.

3. Add the chicken and brown each side for around 4-5 minutes. Place to one side.

4. Add the onion to the pan and fry until soft.

5. Add the garlic, prawns, Cajun seasoning, and red pepper to the pan and cook for around 5 minutes or until prawns become opaque.

6. Add the white rice along with the chopped bell pepper, chicken, and chicken stock to the pan.

7. Cover the pan and allow to simmer for around 25 minutes or until the rice is soft.

8. Serve and enjoy!

Nutrition: Calories: 557 kcal Protein: 18.96 g Fat: 12.34 g Carbohydrates: 93.28 g

Onion, Kale and White Bean Soup

Preparation Time: 15 minutes

Cooking Time: 25 minutes

Servings: 4

Ingredients:

- ¼ cup extra-virgin olive oil
- 1 large onion, thinly sliced
- 2 garlic cloves, thinly sliced
- 1 teaspoon salt
- ¼ teaspoon freshly ground black pepper
- ⅛ Teaspoon red pepper flakes (optional)
- 3 cups stemmed kale leaves cut into ½-inch pieces
- 4 cups vegetable broth
- 1 (15½-ounce) can white beans, drained and rinsed
- 1 teaspoon finely chopped fresh rosemary

Directions:

1. In a huge pot, heat the oil on high heat.

2. Reduce the heat to medium, and add the onion, garlic, salt, pepper, and red pepper flakes (if using). Sauté until the onion is golden, about 10 minutes.

3. Add the kale, and sauté until wilted, 1 to 2 minutes.

4. Pour the broth then bring to a boil.

5. Reduce the heat to simmer, and cook until the kale is soft about 5 minutes.

6. Add the beans and rosemary. Cook until the beans are warmed through at least 2 to 3 minutes and serve.

Nutrition: Calories: 285 Total Fat: 15g Total Carbohydrates: 28g Sugar: 3g Fiber: 9g Protein: 13g

Adobo Lime Chicken Mix

Preparation Time: 10 minutes

Cooking Time: 40 minutes

Servings: 6

Ingredients:

- 6 chicken thighs
- Salt and black pepper to the taste
- 1 tablespoon olive oil
- Zest of 1 lime
- 1½ teaspoons chipotle peppers in adobo sauce
- 1 cup sliced peach
- 1 tablespoon lime juice

Directions:

1.   Warm a pan with the oil on medium-high heat and add the chicken thighs. Season with salt and pepper, then brown for 4 minutes on each side and bake in the oven at 375 degrees F for 20 minutes. In your food processor, mix the peaches with the chipotle, lime zest, and lime juice, then blend and pour over the chicken. Bake for 10 minutes more, divide everything between plates and serve.

2.   Enjoy!

Nutrition: Calories: 309 Fat: 6 Fiber: 4 Carbs: 16 Protein: 15

Mint Zucchini

Preparation Time: 10 minutes

Cooking Time: 7 minutes

Servings: 4

Ingredients:

• 2 tablespoons mint

• 2 zucchinis, halved lengthwise and then slice into half moons

• 1 tablespoon coconut oil, melted

• ½ tablespoon dill, chopped

• A pinch of cayenne pepper

Directions:

1. Heat up a pan with the oil over medium-high heat, add zucchinis, stir and cook for 6 minutes.

2. Add cayenne, dill and mint, stir, cook for 1 minute more, divide between plates and serve.

3. Enjoy!

Nutrition: Calories 46, fat 3,6, fiber 1,3, carbs 3,5, protein 1,3

Phosphorus: 120mg Potassium: 127mg Sodium: 75mg

Sweet Potato and Corn Soup

Preparation Time: 10 minutes

Cooking Time: 20 minutes

Servings: 4

Ingredients:

- ¼ cup extra-virgin olive oil or coconut oil
- 1 medium zucchini, cut into ¼-inch dice
- 1 cup broccoli florets
- 1 cup thinly sliced mushrooms
- 1 small onion, cut into ¼-inch dice
- 4 cups vegetable broth
- 2 cups peeled carrots cut into ¼-inch dice
- 1 cup frozen corn kernels
- 1 cup coconut almond milk or almond milk
- 2 tablespoons finely chopped fresh flat-leaf parsley
- 1 teaspoon salt
- ¼ teaspoon freshly ground black pepper

Directions:

1. In a huge pot, heat the oil on high heat.

2. Add the zucchini, broccoli, mushrooms, and onion and sauté until softened, 5 to 8 minutes.

3. Pour the broth and carrots and place it to a boil.

4. Reduce the heat to a simmer and cook until the carrots are tender, 5 to 7 minutes.

5.	Add the corn, coconut almond milk, parsley, salt, and pepper. Cook on low heat up to the corn is heated through and serve.

Nutrition: Calories: 402 Total Fat: 29g Total Carbohydrates: 31g Sugar: 9g Fiber: 6g Protein: 10g Sodium: 1406mg

Snack

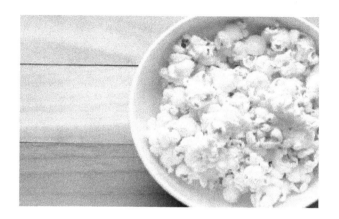

Pumpkin-Turmeric Latte

Preparation time: 10 minutes

Cooking time: 10 minutes

Servings: 1

Ingredients:

- ½ cup brewed espresso or 1 cup brewed strong coffee
- ¼ cup pumpkin purée
- 1 teaspoon vanilla extract
- 1 teaspoon sugar
- ½ teaspoon ground turmeric
- ½ teaspoon ground cinnamon, plus more if needed
- 1 cup 1% almond milk

Directions:

1. Combine the espresso, pumpkin, vanilla, sugar, turmeric, and cinnamon in a medium saucepan over medium heat, whisking occasionally.

2. Warm the almond milk over low heat in a small pan. When it is warm (not hot), whisk it vigorously (or mix with a blender or handheld frother) to make it foamy.

3. Pour the hot coffee mixture into a mug, then top with the frothy almond milk. Sprinkle with more cinnamon, if desired.

Nutrition: Calories: 169; Total Fat: 3g; Saturated Fat: 2g; Cholesterol: 12mg; Sodium: 128mg; Carbohydrates: 26g; Fiber: 3g; Added Sugars: 5g; Protein: 9g; Potassium: 665mg; Vitamin K: 11mcg

Marinated Berries

Preparation time: 5 minutes

Cooking time: 30 minutes

Servings: 4

Ingredients:

- 2 cups fresh strawberries, hulled and quartered
- 1 cup fresh blueberries (optional)
- 2 tablespoons sugar
- 1 tablespoon balsamic vinegar
- 2 tablespoons chopped fresh mint (optional)
- ⅛ teaspoon freshly ground black pepper

Directions:

1. Gently toss the strawberries, blueberries (if using), sugar, vinegar, mint (if using), and pepper in a large nonreactive bowl.

2. Let the flavors blend for at least 25 minutes, or as long as 2 hours.

Nutrition: Calories: 73; Total Fat: 8g; Saturated Fat: 8g; Cholesterol: 0mg; Sodium: 4mg; Carbohydrates: 18g; Fiber: 2g; Added Sugars: 6g; Protein: 1g; Potassium: 162mg; Vitamin K: 9mcg

Dark Hot Chocolate

Preparation time: 5 minutes

Cooking time: 5 minutes

Servings: 2

Ingredients:

- 1¾ cups vanilla soy almond milk
- 1-ounce dark chocolate (70% cacao or more), broken into small pieces

Directions:

1. Heat the soy almond milk in a small saucepan over medium-high heat and add the chocolate. When the almond milk starts bubbling, turn the heat to low.

2. Whisk until the chocolate is melted and fully incorporated. Tip the pot to make sure there is no remaining chocolate on the bottom.

Nutrition: Calories: 149; Total Fat: 8g; Saturated Fat: 3g; Cholesterol: 0mg; Sodium: 105mg; Carbohydrates: 14g; Fiber: 2g; Added Sugars: 5g; Protein: 6g; Potassium: 351mg; Vitamin K: 4mcg

Chickpea Fatteh

Preparation time: 25 minutes

Cooking time: 25 minutes

Servings: 8

Ingredients:

- 2 (4-inch) whole-wheat pitas
- 4 tablespoons extra-virgin olive oil, divided
- 1 (15-ounce) can no-salt-added chickpeas, rinsed and drained
- ⅓ cup pine nuts
- 1 cup plain 1% yogurt
- 2 garlic cloves, minced
- ¼ teaspoon salt
- ½ cup pomegranate seeds (optional)

Directions:

1. Preheat the oven to 375°F.

2. Cut the pitas into 1-inch squares (no need to separate the two halves), and toss with 2 tablespoons of oil in a large bowl. Spread onto a rimmed baking sheet and bake, occasionally shaking the sheet until golden brown, about 10 minutes.

3. Meanwhile, gently warm the chickpeas and 1 tablespoon of oil in a small saucepan over medium-low heat, 4 to 5 minutes.

4.   Toast the pine nuts in a skillet with the remaining 1 tablespoon of oil over medium heat until golden brown, 4 to 5 minutes.

5.   Mix the yogurt with the garlic and salt in a small bowl.

6.   Transfer the toasted pitas to a wide serving bowl. Top with the chickpeas. Drizzle with the yogurt mixture, then top with the pine nuts and pomegranate seeds (if using).

Nutrition: Calories: 198; Total Fat: 12g; Saturated Fat: 2g; Cholesterol: 2mg; Sodium: 144mg; Carbohydrates: 18g; Fiber: 3g; Added Sugars: 0g; Protein: 6g; Potassium: 236mg; Vitamin K: 9mcg

Dark Chocolate and Cherry Trail Mix

Preparation time: 5 minutes

Cooking time: 5 minutes

Servings: Makes 3 cups (¼ cup per serving)

Ingredients:

- 1 cup unsalted almonds
- ⅔ cup dried cherries
- ½ cup walnuts
- ½ cup sweet cinnamon-roasted chickpeas
- ¼ cup dark chocolate chips

Directions:

1. Combine the almonds, cherries, walnuts, chickpeas, and chocolate chips in an airtight container.

2. Store at room temperature for up to 1 week or in the freezer for up to 3 months.

Nutrition: Calories: 174; Total Fat: 12g; Saturated Fat: 2g; Cholesterol: 0mg; Sodium: 18mg; Carbohydrates: 16g; Fiber: 4g; Added Sugars: 7g; Protein: 5g; Potassium: 134mg; Vitamin K: 0mcg

Dessert

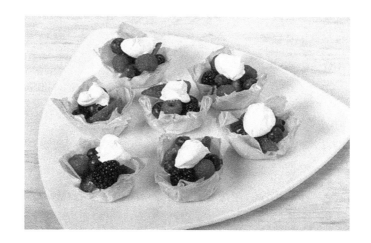

Vanilla Custard

Preparation Time: 7 minutes

Cooking Time: 10 minutes

Servings: 10

Ingredients

- Egg – 1
- Vanilla – 1/8 Teaspoon
- Nutmeg – 1/8 Teaspoon
- Almond Almond Milk – ½ Cup
- Stevia - 2 Tablespoon

Directions

1. Scald The Almond Milk Then Let It Cool Slightly.

2. Break The Egg Into A Bowl And Beat It With The Nutmeg.

3. Add The Scalded Almond Milk, The Vanilla, And The Sweetener To Taste. Mix Well.

4. Place The Bowl In A Baking Pan Filled With ½ Deep Of Water.

5. Bake For 30 Minutes At 325F.

6. Serve.

Nutrition: Calories: 167.3 Fat: 9g Carb: 11g Phosphorus: 205mg Potassium: 249mg Sodium: 124mg Protein: 10g

Lemon-lime Sherbet

Preparation time: 5 minutes, plus 3 hours chilling time

Cooking time: 15 minutes

Servings: 2

Ingredients:

- 2 cups water
- 1 cup granulated sugar
- 3 tablespoons lemon zest, divided
- ½ cup freshly squeezed lemon juice
- Zest of 1 lime
- Juice of 1 lime
- ½ cup heavy (whipping) cream

Directions:

1. Place a large saucepan over medium-high heat and add the water, sugar, and 2 tablespoons of the lemon zest.

2. Bring the mixture to a boil and then reduce the heat and simmer for 15 minutes.

3. Transfer the mixture to a large bowl and add the remaining 1 tablespoon lemon zest, the lemon juice, lime zest, and lime juice.

4. Chill the mixture in the fridge until completely cold, about 3 hours.

5. Whisk in the heavy cream and transfer the mixture to an ice cream maker.

6. Freeze according to the manufacturer's instructions.

Nutrition: Calories: 151; Fat: 6g; Carbohydrates: 26g; Phosphorus: 10mg; Potassium: 27mg; Sodium: 6mg; Protein: 0g

Tart Apple Granita

Preparation time: 15 minutes, plus 4 hours freezing time

Cooking time: 0

Servings: 4

Ingredients:

- ½ cup granulated sugar
- ½ cup water
- 2 cups unsweetened apple juice
- ¼ cup freshly squeezed lemon juice

Directions:

1. In a small saucepan over medium-high heat, heat the sugar and water.

2. Bring the mixture to a boil and then reduce the heat to low and simmer for about 15 minutes or until the liquid has reduced by half.

3. Remove the pan from the heat and pour the liquid into a large shallow metal pan.

4. Let the liquid cool for about 30 minutes and then stir in the apple juice and lemon juice.

5. Place the pan in the freezer.

6. After 1 hour, run a fork through the liquid to break up any ice crystals formed. Scrape down the sides as well.

7. Place the pan back in the freezer and repeat the stirring and scraping every 20 minutes, creating slush.

8. Serve when the mixture is completely frozen and looks like crushed ice, after about 3 hours.

Nutrition: Calories: 157; Fat: 0g; Carbohydrates: 0g; Phosphorus: 10mg; Potassium: 141mg; Sodium: 5mg; Protein: 0g

Pavlova with Peaches

Preparation time: 30 minutes

Cooking time: 1 hour, plus cooling time

Servings: 3

Ingredients:

- 4 large egg whites, at room temperature
- ½ teaspoon cream of tartar
- 1 cup superfine sugar
- ½ teaspoon pure vanilla extract
- 2 cups peaches

Directions:

1. Preheat the oven to 225°F.

2. Line a baking sheet with parchment paper; set aside.

3. In a large bowl, beat the egg whites for about 1 minute or until soft peaks form.

4. Beat in the cream of tartar.

5. Add the sugar, 1 tablespoon at a time, until the egg whites are very stiff and glossy. Do not overbeat.

6. Beat in the vanilla.

7. Evenly spoon the meringue onto the baking sheet so that you have 8 rounds.

8. Use the back of the spoon to create an indentation in the middle of each round.

9. Bake the meringues for about 1 hour or until a light brown crust forms.

10.   Turn off the oven and let the meringues stand, still in the oven, overnight.

11.   Remove the meringues from the sheet and place them on serving plates.

12.   Spoon the peaches, dividing evenly, into the centers of the meringues, and serve.

13.   Store any unused meringues in a sealed container at room temperature for up to 1 week.

Nutrition: Calories: 132; Fat: 0g; Carbohydrates: 32g; Phosphorus: 7mg; Potassium: 95mg; Sodium: 30mg; Protein: 2g

Tropical Vanilla Snow Cone

Preparation time: 15 minutes, plus freezing time

Cooking time: 0

Servings: 2

Ingredients:

- 1 cup pineapple
- 1 cup frozen strawberries
- 6 tablespoons water
- 2 tablespoons granulated sugar
- 1 tablespoon vanilla extract

Directions:

1.   In a large saucepan, mix the peaches, pineapple, strawberries, water, and sugar over medium-high heat and bring to a boil.

2.   Reduce the heat to low and simmer the mixture, stirring occasionally, for 15 minutes.

3.   Remove from the heat and let the mixture cool completely, for about 1 hour.

4.   Stir in the vanilla and transfer the fruit mixture to a food processor or blender.

5.   Purée until smooth, and pour the purée into a 9-by-13-inch glass baking dish.

6.   Cover and place the dish in the freezer overnight.

7.   When the fruit mixture is completely frozen, use a fork to scrape the sorbet until you have flaked flavored ice.

8. Scoop the ice flakes into 4 serving dishes.

Nutrition: Calories: 92; Fat: 0g; Carbohydrates: 22g; Phosphorus: 17mg; Potassium: 145mg; Sodium: 4mg; Protein: 1g

Apple Crunch Pie

Preparation Time: 10 minutes

Cooking Time: 35 minutes

Servings: 8

Ingredients

- 4 large tart apples, peeled, seeded and sliced
- ½ cup of white all-purpose flour
- ⅓ cup margarine
- 1 cup of sugar
- ¾ cup of rolled oat flakes
- ½ teaspoon of ground nutmeg

Directions

1. Preheat the oven to 375F/180C.
2. Place the apples over a lightly greased square pan (around 7 inches).
3. Mix the rest of the ingredients in a medium bowl with and spread the batter over the apples.
4. Bake for 30-35 minutes or until the top crust has gotten golden brown.
5. Serve hot.

Nutrition: Calories: 261.9 kcal Carbohydrate: 47.2 g Protein: 1.5 g Sodium: 81 mg Potassium: 123.74 mg Phosphorus: 35.27 mg

Dietary Fiber: 2.81 g Fat: 7.99 g

CPSIA information can be obtained
at www.ICGtesting.com
Printed in the USA
BVHW041410160421
605143BV00014B/1476